Nude

unveiling your inner beauty & sensuality

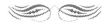

Kym Jackson and Theresa Roemer

authorHOUSE®

AuthorHouse™
1663 Liberty Drive
Bloomington, IN 47403
www.authorhouse.com
Phone: 1-800-839-8640

First published by AuthorHouse 04/18/2011
ISBN: 978-1-4567-6242-1 (e)
ISBN: 978-1-4567-6240-7 (dj)
ISBN: 978-1-4567-6241-4 (sc)
Library of Congress Control Number: 2011906059

Printed in the United States of America

Any people depicted in stock imagery provided by iStock are models, and such images are being used for illustrative purposes only. Certain stock imagery © iStock.

This book is printed on acid-free paper.

Edited by Anne Dejoie-Lucas
Nefatari Cooper, Contributing Editor

Cover design and NUDE Logo by:
Lauren Designs, www.laurendesigns.com

Photos by:
Ladd Photography, www.laddphotography.com
Tracy Hicks Photography, www.tracyhicksphotography.com

www.experiencenude.com

Inside quotes and tidbits adapted from randomhistory.com and random facts.

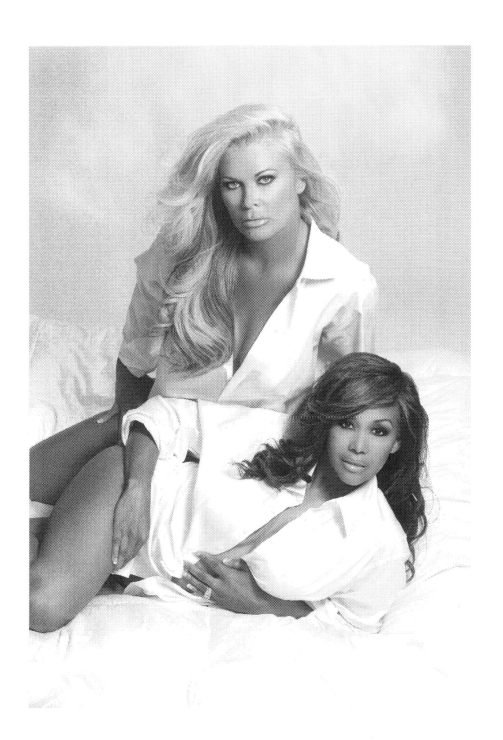

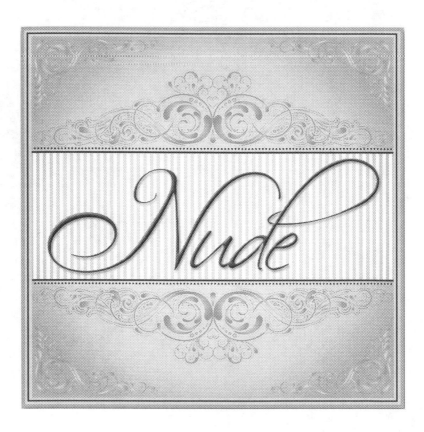

Nude

This book is dedicated to our loving husbands,
Willard and Lamar, who encourage us,
support us, and love us unconditionally.

Contents

Foreword   xi

Acknowledgments   xiii

Chapter 1   The Language of Nude   1

Chapter 2   Flirtatious Fitness   7

Chapter 3   Nutrition for the Mind and Body   19

Chapter 4   Tantalizing Talk, In and Out of the Bedroom   33

Chapter 5   Getting Ready for That "Good Good"   43

Chapter 6   Let the Bedroom Games Begin   49

Chapter 7   Revving Up for Round Two   61

Chapter 8   Recipe for a Yummy Sexual Relationship   69

Chapter 9   Spring-Clean Your Sex Life   75

Chapter 10   Keep It Hot, and Keep It Coming   81

About the Authors   85

People who invest themselves in being what they can be and, even more importantly, people who invest themselves in helping others be what they can be, are involved in the single most important work on this earth.

Eric Hoffer

Foreword

Close your eyes and imagine for a minute what it would feel like to just "let go"! To enjoy every aspect of your life, without worrying about anything. Without letting your inhibitions hold you back. Just letting go and taking your romantic life to the next level, where you unleash, unveil, and uncover beauty and sensuality without holding back. *Nude: Unveiling Your Inner Beauty and Sensuality* helps guide you to that wonderful destination, where you understand how fitness, nutrition, hormones, intimacy, beauty, sex appeal, confidence, and sensuality all flow together to create harmony within yourself and with your partner. Whether you're exercising together, hiking or biking, relaxing at the spa, or just doing chores around the house, every minute you spend together can be spent strengthening your relationship and keeping it hot, spicy, sensual, and romantic. Just turn the pages and see what sexy little secrets lie within … Enjoy!

It's not what we have in our life but who we have in our life that counts.

—Unknown

Acknowledgments

from Kym …

First, I would like to thank our Heavenly Father for his guidance and patience. Thank you also to my beautiful family and friends for the love and support you have given me.

My mom, Elouise, has been my constant source of strength and my biggest fan ever since I can remember. I'm truly grateful that God blessed me with her as my mother. I love you unconditionally!

To Will, Blake, Mary, and Chauncey, may you never stop reaching for your hopes and dreams. I love you with all my heart and soul!

Cookie and Carol, you mean the world to me! Mirna, you're so invaluable to me. Sheila and Kristin, thanks for helping us put our best "faces" forward! Your love and support mean the world to me! Cassandra, Shirelle, Karen and Kena!

Anne, thank you for your kindness and support. You have helped shape our thoughts and bring them to life!

Theresa, my co-author and "BFF," unveiling this book with you has been a whirlwind of excitement! Big huggies!!!

My husband, my friend, my lover, Willard, you are my dream come true! After twenty-six years, it still feels like yesterday that we began our love affair. Thanks you for being open to my dreams. Passionately … I love you, Sweetheart. The best is yet to come …

from Theresa ...

I want to sincerely thank those who have helped shape my life. There are more of you than I could possibly acknowledge. This book's very existence is the culmination of friendships and support of many individuals who have impacted my professional and personal journey, and I am profoundly grateful to each of you.

First, I would like to thank my Heavenly Father, who has given me the strength and faith to get through the adversities that have been tossed into my life. I would also like to thank my son, Michael, and my brother, Brian, who are looking down on me from heaven, for giving me the courage to pursue my dreams and make them come true.

I would definitely like to thank my wonderful, loving husband, Lamar, for his constant love, devotion, and support in letting me be whatever I want to be in this life. With you by my side, I can achieve anything!

Thanks to my daughter, Tashina, my parents, my siblings, my stepchildren, and my extended family for their continued support and for believing in me through all that I have been and all that I am yet to become.

I also want to thank Kym, my friend who co-authored this book. Your support, friendship, and willingness to think outside the box help to inspire me to reach beyond what is—toward what can be.

Last, but not least, I am especially grateful to our editor, Anne Lucas, for your ability to take our words and thoughts and give them life on the page.

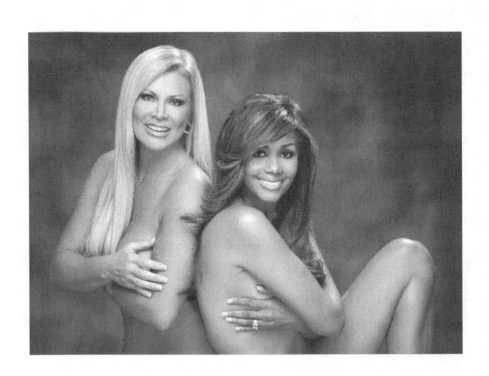

Sex appeal is fifty percent what you've got and fifty percent what people think you've got.

Sophia Loren

Chapter One

The Language of Nude

Ever been nude? Sure you have! In reality, it's the essence of who you are. It's how you came into this world, and it's what is revealed when you open up and let down the curtains of security and comfort that all of us too often like to hide behind. Time and again, as two seasoned pageant participants, we step onstage in front of judges and thousands of people and rise to the occasion. We're dressed to perfection, our makeup is timeless, our smiles are radiant, and we say and do all the right things that we know need to be said and done to win a pageant. That same confidence we take to the pageants is also brought to our relationships. When you step into the bedroom, you should know that you are looking fabulous, smelling wonderful, and radiating sexiness. Use that same confidence to deliver what your spouse needs so you can reach blissful ecstasy together. After all, our husbands love us unconditionally and aren't judging us the way pageant judges are, so why should we hold back with them? This is the time to be really "nude" and bare all—feelings, emotions, passion, romance!

Oftentimes, the word *nude* conjures up negative connotations of XXX-rated, "behind closed doors," pornographic behavior. However, to show your partner the "nude" you is to unveil and discover everything there is to know about you. Not just the physical nudity of your body, but also the unraveling of your innermost thoughts and ideas, the revelation of beauty deep within, the rough diamond waiting to be polished with intimacy and romance—the total you! Hot and sexy comes in all ages, sizes, and colors. Don't let a good sex life die out or pass you by! The last time we checked, orgasms had no expiration date or prerequisites!

We recently had the pleasure of traveling together with our husbands to the captivating French Riviera. One night, as we sat by the beach listening to the waves crash against the rocks and the sensuality whisper all around us in the refreshing, exhilarating night air, we began sharing stories about some of the things that we felt made our relationships so very special and exciting. As we shared romantic epics of passion, healthy lifestyles, intimacy, exercise routines, and much, much more, it became clear to us that we needed to share our sexy little secrets with other women who want to embrace their strength, inner beauty, and sensuality. Women need to know the power they possess to make their own relationships as fulfilling and erotic as we try to make our own. Our husbands were in total agreement and gave us the go-ahead to tell our stories. Over the next chapters, we'll share with you how we stay in shape, stay motivated, try to stay sexy, and most importantly, stay positive. *Nude* is your how-to guide to keep the feeling of being sensual inside and out. Within these pages are our own experiences and secrets, and we hope this book inspires you to unleash, unveil, and partake in some "nudity" of your own as you embark on a discovery of the "total you"!

Sharing the world of pageants, we've both held titles for various beauty pageant competitions and have become comfortable wearing the title of "beauty queen." But we also wear the titles of mother, wife, daughter, grandmother, and businesswoman. Above all of those these, however, we wear the title of "woman"—one who is distinctively feminine in nature, a characteristic that is unique. While we are all unique, many women share an experimental curiosity and a need for passionate intimacy in the bedroom, which also appears in our everyday lives.

We have talked to so many ladies who say they no longer feel sexy. They've gained some weight, noticed a few crow's feet and gray hair, or just don't have the same energy they used to. On the other hand, some women simply have not yet discovered what makes them sexy. The good news is that the ability to feel and exude *sexy* is within your control. Diet and exercise, hair color, and a good doctor can all determine your level of sexy. We have to accent the positives in our lives and play down our "not so great" attributes. Be you and do you! Don't feel as though you have to explain to anybody why you do what you do—hair, makeup, extensions, weight. You make the decisions that are most comfortable for you and your partner.

Even as we get older, we know we can hold our own against

any woman. However, it's not a competition, and we've learned to love every age that we've been blessed to experience so far! We look the best that we can and feel fabulous! We recognize that we're not perfect, but that doesn't stop us from radiating the self-confidence, self-esteem, and sexiness that all women should embrace within themselves—fully clothed or baring it all! After all, what have you got to hide?

The more we pondered that thought, the more we came to realize the title and theme for this book. *Nude* means to open up, first to yourself and then to your partner. Learn to love yourself completely. Believe us, everyone has insecurities, but it's how they are handled that makes some people seem like they are free of inhibitions. Don't allow insecurities to regulate your life. Manage your well-being with maturity and sensibility, and give your best in everything you do in life. When it comes down to determining what makes a relationship strong, one thing is certain: it needs intimacy … sexual intimacy, intellectual and mental intimacy, emotional intimacy, social intimacy, and spiritual intimacy. Before you can comfortably flow into the romance and sensuality of a relationship, it's important to first come into your own comfort zone by facing up to who you are and who you want to present to your partner. With this realization comes learning about your body from the inside out—hormones, nutrition, fitness, and self-esteem—and then finding out how these things actually affect what you bring to the table in the relationship. Knowing how and when to flirt, communicating with your partner, overcoming inhibitions, and embracing your true self play major roles in being all your partner wants and needs in a mate. *Nude: Unveiling Your Inner*

Beauty and Sensuality identifies vital tips you need to know to keep it hot and keep it coming, night after night, year after year.

Naked Truth: Women who read romance novels have sex twice as often as those who don't!

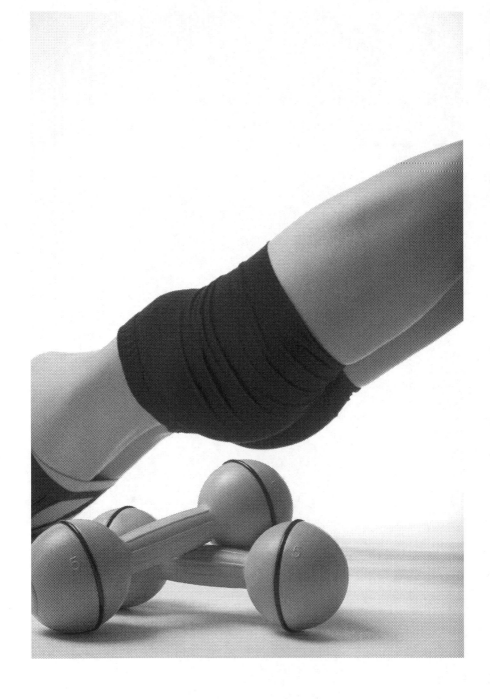

Confidence is the sexiest thing a woman can have. It's much sexier than any body part.

Aimee Mullins

Chapter Two

Flirtatious Fitness

Sex appeal!!! Just what is it about sex appeal that you don't understand? Everyone wants it, and with a healthy mind-set, everyone can achieve it! There's no golden rule that says you have to be five foot seven and a size 4 to be sexy. There is, however, an unspoken understanding that healthiness is a must for sexiness. Whatever your size, it's important that you have a healthy attitude, healthy lifestyle, and healthy atmosphere around you. These build confidence, and confidence emits sexiness, for petite and plus-size women alike. Being healthy is the sexiest thing you can do for your body—mentally, physically, and spiritually. It's important to make the best of your assets ... to stay youthful and healthy-looking, be in reasonably good shape, and maintain a positive, uplifting attitude and outlook on life. These add to increased confidence and energy, not just for your sex life, but for life as a whole. Routine workouts release "feel-good" chemicals into your system and help to improve your self-esteem as well as your shape. That "feel-good" high can easily trickle over into your sex life as well.

Let's face it: it's hard to feel sexy when you are out of shape, depressed, or have low self-esteem. Just as happiness comes from within, so does sexiness. No one else can do this for you. You have to start today—right now—to set the goals you want to reach. Nutrition, exercise, and hormones … imagine that! Those three ingredients influence weight, mood swings, energy levels, and believe it or not, sensuality. Who feels sensual and sexy when she's tired, depressed, and unhealthy?

It's amazing how hormones work to control so much of what goes on in the body—everything from blood sugar to energy, fat metabolism, muscle maintenance, moods, and sex drive. In fact, it's been proven that hormones have the following effects on the body:

- stimulation or inhibition of growth
- mood swings
- activation or inhibition of the immune system
- regulation of metabolism
- preparation of the body for mating, fighting, fleeing, and other activity
- preparation of the body for a new phase of life, such as puberty, parenting, and menopause
- control of the reproductive cycle
- hunger cravings

A woman's hormones control just about every aspect of her body, and anyone exposed to high levels of stress should consult a doctor to make sure there are no hormone imbalances that could be affecting fitness, health, and more. Stress raises levels of cortisol, which causes hormone imbalances, decreases testosterone, and increases facial hair and weight gain around the waistline. The good news is that you can help to prevent these imbalances by eating well-balanced, nutritious, healthy meals. Through proper diet and exercise, you can manipulate and once again become the boss of your hormones so you can feel great. Get your sexy back!

We truly live by the belief that "If you have your health, you have your wealth!" When we came into this world, God gave each of us a body to treat as a temple. It's not to be abused and neglected. We are taught as children to brush our teeth daily to keep them healthy. Shouldn't the same daily care and attention be given to our bodies? Here's another scenario. If you're having a home built, wouldn't you want the best builder? You'd want the nicest natural floors, the greatest electronics and appliances, and the best insurance coverage available. You'd spend time each week cleaning, decorating, and manicuring the lawn, in order to make it appealing both inside and out. So how can we put that much effort into a house and not be willing to put the same into our bodies? Many people don't get regular health checkups, they eat poorly, and they make up excuses as to why they can't exercise. Our bodies have to last a lifetime; we don't have the option to trade them in like cars, or sell them like homes when we're ready to upgrade. Doesn't it stand to reason that we should put more emphasis on our fleshly building than we do on the physical building or home we purchase? Let's get excited about cleansing, decorating, and maintaining our bodies as we do our homes and cars. It's as easy as a personal routine of thirty to sixty minutes a day, three to four days a week, which includes weight training, walking, jogging, dancing, cycling, aerobics, spinning, golfing, push-ups, crunches, and any combination of these and more to help mold you into the healthy person you desire to be. Try starting each day with a simple twenty-minute warm-up like a brisk walk outside or on a treadmill.

Want to further enhance your workouts? Then try the following as part of a full six-day weekly regimen. Divide the body into four parts:

1. shoulders/abs
2. legs
3. back/biceps
4. chest/triceps

Work one part each day for four of your six workout days; add cardio to your routine the other two days. Building muscle not only helps to mold your body but also increases your metabolism, which helps you burn fat quicker.

Here's a simple six-day plan that you can try:

(By the way, you can use the Internet to learn the proper techniques/procedures for doing most of these exercises.)

Day 1 – Best Chest/Tantalizing Triceps
- Warm-up – 60 jumping jacks
- Dumbbell press – 20 repetitions/3 times
- Dumbbell flyer – 20 repetitions/3 times
- Close-hand push-ups – 20 repetitions/3 times
- Reverse kickbacks – 20 repetitions/3 times

- Head bangers (dumbbell) – 20 repetitions/3 times
- Dips – 20 repetitions/3 times

Day 2 – Long Legs/Flat Abs

- Warm-up – knee-ups, 1 minute
- Lunges – 1 minute/3 times
- Sissy squats with weights – 20 repetitions/3 times
- Dumbbell dead lifts – 20 repetitions/3 times
- Plyometrics jump side to side – 20 repetitions/3 times
- Dumbbell front squats – 20 repetitions/3 times
- Bicycle (abs) – 1 minute/3 times
- Crossover crunches – 1 minute/3 times

Day 3 – Sizzling Cardio

- Brisk walk, jogging, aerobic exercise, at least 30 minutes

Day 4 – Sexy Back/Beautiful Biceps

- Warm-up – knee-ups, 1 minute
- Wide dumbbell pulls – 20 repetitions/3 times
- Alternating dumbbell – 20 repetitions/3 times
- Pull-ups – 20 repetitions/3 times
- Alternating curls with rotation – 20 repetitions/3 times
- Hammer curls – 20 repetitions/3 times
- Single curls – 20 repetitions/3 times

Day 5 – Sensual Shoulders/Tight Abs

- Warm-up – 60 jumping jacks
- Side dumbbell raises – 20 repetitions/3 times
- Shoulder presses – 20 repetitions/3 times

- Front dumbbell raises – 20 repetitions/3 times
- Bent-over flyers – 20 repetitions/3 times
- V-tucks with dumbbell – 1 minute/3 times
- Reverse crunches – 1 minute/3 times

Day 6 – Sizzling Cardio
- Brisk walk, jogging, aerobic exercise – at least 30 minutes

Day 7 – Rest Your Body!!

To avoid burnout and damage to the muscles, your body needs a day each week to rest. If you're not a member of a gym or spa, most, if not all, of these exercises can easily be done at home. There are several books and websites available that can show you additional exercises to start toning and shaping each of these areas. Don't forget to also do your Kegel exercises every day. For best results, empty your bladder, relax and squeeze the pelvic floor muscles with intensity, holding it three to five seconds for each Kegel. You can do these just about anytime, anywhere, and nobody will know you're working hard to keep things nice, tight, and just right!

Women spend thousands of dollars on clothes, shoes, hair, manicures, pedicures, waxes, extensions, wigs, lifts, tucks, and other external enhancements to "look nice," yet they won't opt for putting a little extra effort into their fitness and nutrition program for free each week to look and feel healthy. They gravitate toward instant gratification, which comes much more easily than putting forth the time to change routines and transform the body from the inside out. Don't get discouraged if you don't see an immediate change. Smart lifestyle changes are gradual and permanent, and you'll reap rewards that aren't for sale in any store or salon.

We want you to learn to be as dedicated to your health as you are to your jobs and your families, because without your health, you have nothing! Being healthy and feeling well doesn't have to cost a lot or be confusing. They are simple, but take dedication and commitment, just like having a healthy relationship.

Always remember, ladies, fitness doesn't have to be a solitary adventure! Sometimes we get so busy being coworkers, students, mothers, and entrepreneurs, we forget how to be girlfriends and wives. Busy schedules and parenthood can lead to less time for intimacy. If we become overweight and out of shape, the end result can be devastating to a healthy intimate relationship. That's why working out with your partner is a good form of foreplay. Caressing each other's firm, tight bodies while stretching before a good workout is a great way to let your partner know what's in store later. And who wouldn't enjoy watching their partner's body move through its gyrations while doing crunches or push-ups? Be honest. When your partner is doing push-ups, don't you fantasize about just easing in underneath and letting nature take over? What better foreplay than to straddle-stretch together … sitting opposite each other, legs spread wide apart, with nothing between the two of you except for thoughts of hot, wild sex. If you really want something fun, try a few stretches at home together—nude! This can lead to one of the best forms of exercise there is—sex! Burn some calories together by spending a day cleaning and cooking, but do it nude! Just imagine!!! You might not get all the dusting finished, but no doubt you'll both get a really good workout before the day is done!

Here are some more romantic suggestions to help you stay in shape together:

- Do stomach crunches while holding each other's legs.
- Spot for each other during weight lifting. The view from a press bench can be quite stimulating if your partner stands in the right place!
- Do cardio walking, one behind the other. Who doesn't like looking at a sexy bottom moving rhythmically in front of him or her?
- Swim together and take time between laps to embrace and caress each other in the water—very stimulating! If possible, try skinny-dipping! You'll love it!!!
- Count for each other during your workout sets.
- Play your favorite romantic, sexual music while working out together at home.
- Pump each other up with sweet words and bedroom talk while working out.
- Do yard work together. Make sure the neighbors aren't watching as you bend over in front of your partner to pull weeds.
- Grab a hula hoop and start sweating! It's great fun and also provides an excellent core and ab workout. Make it fun for your partner too. If you're really good at hula-hooping, try alternating the speed and turning rhythmically so your partner can watch you gyrating from the front, the back, and the sides. He can watch all parts of you moving in various ways.

If you're really creative and have good hoop control, see if you can slowly remove your shirt while still hula-hooping and see what your partner's reaction will be!

Get excited about exercise, and try something different so it doesn't get boring. Ask a friend about the *Kama Sutra*, or check online to learn more ways to increase your pleasure and stir things up with exciting new positions that you can do all around the home, including the bathtub, staircase, and laundry room. You'd be surprised what you can do with regular household items like metal spoons and spatulas, which stimulate nipples and are ideal for light spanking.

Another trendy new form of exercise is the use of stripper poles. Guys enjoy watching women work their stuff at the strip club, so why not get your own pole and keep him home? It also provides a great cardio workout. Try it; you'll both like it! We both tried it, and we loved it! It felt a bit strange and awkward at first, but then as our husbands responded, we become more comfortable and had more fun. We also quickly discovered that pageant shoes are great for the bedroom! Made similar to the shoes pole dancers and exotic dancers wear, they have clear Lucite heels and decorative embellished tops. Not only are they comfortable, but they're also easy to find, as most bridal stores and popular shoe stores carry them, and they are a perfect complement to that sexy lingerie you've got tucked away!

No longer just for exotic club dancers, pole-stripper–style workouts are showing up at many dance studios and gyms as an exciting alternative for women to get in shape while gaining confidence and getting in touch with the sensual side of things.

This combination of dancing and gymnastics involves dancing sensually with a vertical pole. It is now recognized as a form of exercise that can be used as both an aerobic and anaerobic workout, for both women and men. How enticing for your spouse to watch you working out at a pole studio!! It can be such a turn-on for both of you if you play your cards right!!

The popular Internet site Wikipedia defines a couple of popular pole styles. The standard dance pole typically consists of a hollow steel or brass pole with a circular cross section, running from floor to ceiling. The diameter is usually around five centimeters (two inches), allowing it to be gripped comfortably with one hand.

Another common pole is the spinning pole; as its name suggests, it is similar to a standard dance pole but spins using ball bearings. The purpose of this pole is to create better momentum and higher rates of speed, in order to have a greater dramatic effect. Home versions are available that may be used for practice or aerobic exercise. Poles can be composed of polished stainless steel, chromed steel, brass, powder coating, or titanium coating. Poles also can be made of acrylic glass, which allows the use of "glow poles" with LED lighting effects. Each material surface has different gripping properties. Polished steel is one of the slickest materials, which provides for a faster, more fluid dance; brass poles provide more friction, allowing for an easier hold with hands or thighs and creating a slow, sensual dance style. A pole can be held in place by using threading to brace it against a ceiling joist. There are also poles that do not require construction and can be set up using tension. Stationary, rotating, and switchable versions are available. Portable and permanent poles come in various lengths, colors, and styles and help to bring the fantasy home for you and your partner. Enjoy striptease aerobics in the privacy of your own home while you get the firm, toned body that the dancers boast. Poles are great fun and also offer a workout that results in

- increased upper body strength
- toned abs and core
- building up of upper leg muscles
- increased flexibility
- increased self-esteem as a result of body control

Of course, what pole dance would be complete without an unforgettable, seductive lap dance! Make sure, however, that you save that part for home and not inside the studio!

Need we say more about where this will lead? Try it; we think you'll love it!

Sexy Fact: Foreplay and sex can burn as much as three hundred calories an hour. An average person can actually burn two hundred calories with just thirty minutes of active sex, and can lose four pounds a year simply by engaging in thirty minutes of sex twice a week.

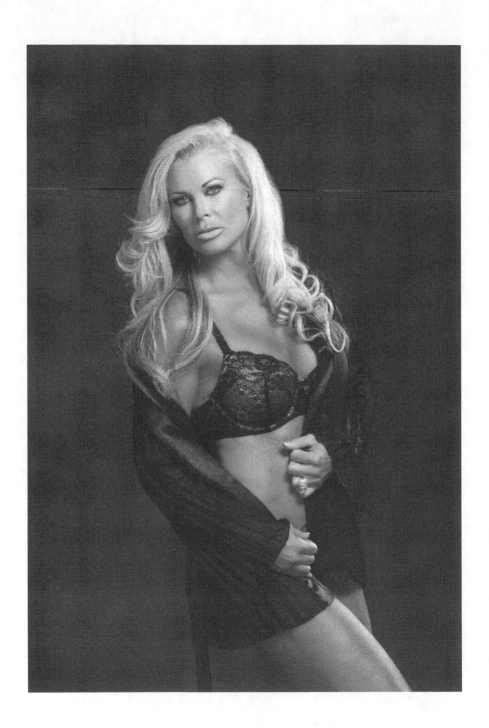

Living a healthy lifestyle will only deprive you of poor health, lethargy, and fat.

Jill Johnson

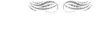

Chapter Three

Nutrition for the Mind and Body

Exercise isn't the only thing needed to maintain good health and peace of mind. Good nutrition also is a key factor. Despite the roadblocks society throws down, healthy eating doesn't have to be a challenge. Fast food can be consumed in a healthy manner, and so can other "forbidden" foods. The keys are proper knowledge and knowing how and when to eat certain foods, and what to do afterward when you do choose to indulge in some of those "forbidden favorites."

Every year we are presented with the daunting task of shaving a few pounds here and there to fit into that perfect hot dress. The pageant world can be very cutthroat, with high demands of sticking to the uniform look of long, lean legs, well-defined arms, and an award-winning smile. (By the way, putting Vaseline on your teeth helps keep your lips from sticking to your teeth.) When you are standing on a stage next to numerous women who all seem to be the perfect "10," it can be very intimidating. Many girls don't eat at all, but starving yourself to death isn't the way. Regardless of that special upcoming event in your life—whether it is a wedding, a class reunion, or in our case a pageant—preparation is the key. We always allow ourselves the proper amount of preparation time so that we are able to be confident not only in how we look but also in how we feel.

Losing weight, inches, and body fat for a pageant or any other event doesn't have to seem like an insurmountable task. It's really not that hard when nutrition is factored in. Your goal is not to aim for skinny, but rather to aim for healthy! Eating well-balanced meals along with following a proper exercise regimen has been proven to be the best way to achieve your goal and maintain *your* sexy, which is different for each woman. You will see later in this chapter The Beauty Queen meal plan that works wonders for us!

You should allow yourself six weeks to realistically obtain your goal. This goal is much easier to reach if you engage in what we call The Buddy System! The Buddy System is a program that requires a partner, such as a personal trainer, girlfriend, neighbor, or spouse, who holds you accountable for your actions. Proper nutrition can be hard to follow without your support system. A dedication to a proper healthy eating plan that includes plenty of fresh fruits and vegetables, fish and chicken, and a willingness to reduce or completely let go of the sweets, high-carbohydrate foods, and alcohol makes all the difference in the world. Much of what should be done is really just common sense.

The first step is to leave the excuses on the shelf. Start now, and make a commitment to stay motivated to reach your goal, however big or small it may seem. Making sure you take the right vitamins and minerals to help supplement your healthy way of eating is also very important, as is drinking plenty of water. Eight to ten glasses of water a day for proper hydration and improved well-being is a vital ingredient to the new healthy you. A few liters a day with fresh squeezed lemon juice will aid in flushing the body of toxins and will help you feel fuller throughout the day, while also burning fat.

It's never too soon to see a nutritionist who can evaluate if you're eating right and taking the right vitamins and supplements to keep your body and your mind in top shape. Imbalanced hormones can affect weight gain, hair loss, fatigue, moodiness, vaginal dryness, libido, sex drive, and more. With new research and increased knowledge in bio-identical hormones, women should understand that they can take control of their health in this area and make changes in order to see improvements in hormonal areas that are lacking.

Immune System and Energy-Boosting Foods

- Garlic—fights infection and bacteria
- Oats and barley—boost immunity, speed wound healing, and may help antibiotics work better
- Yogurt—helps keep stomach and intestines free of disease-causing germs
- Chicken soup—can boost the immune system and fight the common cold
- Tea—full of antioxidants to boost the immune system

(to get up to five times more antioxidants from your tea bag, bob it up and down while you brew)

- Sweet potatoes—have large amounts of beta-carotene, which helps boost vitamin A
- Mushrooms—increase the production and activity of white blood cells

Our secret to getting a hot, healthy body is to eat clean foods that balance your hormones, detox your body, and burn fat. Redefine and rediscover fruits and vegetables. Leave behind the excess sweets, high-carb foods, and abundance of alcohol, which will work against your efforts to detox, cleanse, and streamline your body. Amazingly enough, people don't realize how many calories they consume in liquid beverages, especially alcohol. Alcohol causes your body to pump out more estrogen and less testosterone. Over time, this hormonal imbalance increases the fat in your body. Alcohol not only dehydrates the body, it also strains the liver, which responds by decreasing fat burning.

We suggest you engage the assistance of a nutritionist or dietician to help you start changing your eating habits from not-so-good to great. Not sure how to start? One good suggestion is to make a list of your ten worst dietary vices, and then remove them from your diet one at a time—either one each week, or one each month. But the key is to remove them. Is bread a problem area? Then remove it from your diet. Too much snacking? Then cut regular chips from your diet and change instead to baked chips and eventually fruit. Swap brown rice for white, and corn tortillas for flour. Definitely cut sugar completely, or choose a sugar substitute whenever possible. Small changes will work just as well as drastic ones if you stick to them over a long period of time and convert them into new healthy lifestyle choices.

"I never know how much I'm supposed to eat." Haven't we all tried that excuse before? Trust us; portion control is easier to manage than you might realize. There are simple tricks to measuring servings of various foods. For example, a cup of tossed salad is the amount you can hold in both hands cupped together. A four-ounce serving of protein such as meat or fish is usually the size of the palm of your hand. A cup of cooked grains, veggies, or fruit is about the size of your fist.

We're going to share with you a seven-day plan that can be followed for as few or as many weeks as necessary to reach your goal, whether you're trying to lose ten, thirty, fifty, or even seventy or more pounds. Just remember to also factor in desire, determination, and dedication, and get your physician's approval to make sure this plan won't pose any adverse health effects.

Seven-Day "Beauty Queen" Meal Plan

(Each day represents a daily intake of approximately 1,200 calories.)

Day One:

Breakfast: Don't be afraid to start the day with a cup of coffee. The aroma has been known to act as a natural aphrodisiac that stimulates parts of the brain as well as also stimulating parts of the body. Drink up!

- 1 cup oatmeal (seasoned with a sugar substitute, cinnamon, and vanilla)
- ¼ melon (honeydew or cantaloupe)

Mid-Morning Snack:
- 8-ounce whey protein shake

Lunch:
- Tossed salad
- 1–2 tablespoons salad dressing (lite or fat free, or try a mixture of 1 teaspoon olive oil with 2 tablespoons balsamic vinegar)

Mid-Afternoon Snack:
- 2 hard-boiled eggs

Dinner:
- 4 ounces grilled orange roughy or lean fish
- 1 cup steamed asparagus

Day Two: (Seems new, but keep pushing forward. It will all be worth it!)

Breakfast:
- 1 cup Greek-style or fat-free yogurt
- ¼ melon (honeydew or cantaloupe)

Mid-Morning Snack:
- 1 tablespoon raw almonds
- 1 tablespoon peanut butter, plain or on celery stick

Lunch:
- 1 cup low-sodium lentil soup
- 1 cup tossed salad

- 1–2 tablespoons salad dressing (lite or fat free, or try a mixture of 1 teaspoon olive oil with 2 tablespoons balsamic vinegar or lemon juice)

Mid-Afternoon Snack:
- 8-ounce whey protein shake

Dinner:
- 4 ounces lean ground beef (grilled)
- 1 cup brown rice

Day Three: (Might be a little tough, but hang in there!)

Breakfast:
- 4 ounces lean ground turkey
- 1 banana

Mid-Morning Snack:
- 1 cup low-fat cottage cheese
- 1 apple, peach, or pear

Lunch:
- Tossed salad
- 1–2 tablespoons salad dressing (lite or fat free, or try a mixture of 1 teaspoon olive oil with 2 tablespoons balsamic vinegar)
- 4 ounces skinless chicken breast (grilled)
- 1 slice whole-grain bread

Mid-Afternoon Snack:
- 2 hard-boiled eggs

Dinner:
- 4 ounces grilled halibut or lean fish

- 1 baked sweet potato (seasoned with a sugar substitute, cinnamon, and vanilla)

Day Four: (You should be feeling more comfortable now, and cravings should be subsiding!)

Breakfast:
- 8-ounce whey protein shake
- 1 tablespoon peanut butter, plain or on celery stick

Mid-Morning Snack:
- 2 ounces low-fat mozzarella cheese
- 1 pear, plum, or apple

Lunch:
- 6 ounces water-packed tuna (mixed with 2 tablespoons low-fat or fat-free mayonnaise)
- 1 cup fresh green salad
- 6 whole-grain crackers

Mid-Afternoon Snack:
- 1 large peach or 1 cup green seedless grapes or strawberries

Dinner:
- 4 ounces roasted Cornish hen
- 1 cup winter squash

Day Five: (Your body should be adjusting, and your moods should be balancing out!)

Breakfast:
- 1 cup low-fat cottage cheese

- ½ grapefruit
- 1 slice whole-grain bread, plain or toasted

Mid-Morning Snack:
- 8-ounce whey protein shake

Lunch:
- 1 cup fresh green salad
- 4 ounces boiled shrimp (approximately 6 to 8 medium-size)
- 1–2 tablespoons salad dressing (lite or fat free, or try a mixture of 1 teaspoon olive oil with 2 tablespoons balsamic vinegar)

Mid-Afternoon Snack:
- 1 banana

Dinner:
- 4 ounces grilled lean steak
- 1 cup steamed cauliflower or broccoli
- 1 cup butternut squash (seasoned with cinnamon, allspice, and nutmeg)

Day Six: (By now, you might be able to see a slight weight loss and your confidence should be growing. Keep up the good work; it's paying off!)

Breakfast:
- 1 cup Greek-style or fat-free yogurt
- 1 cup oatmeal (seasoned with a sugar substitute, cinnamon, and vanilla, or cream of wheat)

Mid-Morning Snack:
- 2 tablespoons almonds

Lunch:
- 4 ounces grilled chicken breast

Mid-Afternoon Snack:
- 1 cup fresh chopped fruit

Dinner:
- 4 ounces grilled tilapia or lean fish
- 1 cup steamed green beans
- 1 baked sweet potato (seasoned with a sugar substitute, cinnamon, and vanilla)

Day Seven: (One whole week of clean, healthy eating and transforming your body into a wonderful new you!)

Breakfast:
- 2 scrambled eggs
- 1 cup cream of wheat

Mid-Afternoon Snack:
- 2 tablespoons raw almond butter
- 3 celery sticks

Lunch:
- 1 cup fresh green salad
- 1–2 tablespoons salad dressing (lite or fat free, or try a mixture of 1 teaspoon olive oil with 2 tablespoons balsamic vinegar or lemon juice)
- 4 ounces grilled salmon
- 1 cup chopped vegetables

Mid-Afternoon Snack:

- 2 tablespoons almonds
- 1 apple, pear, or plum

Dinner:
- 4 ounces pork tenderloin (baked or grilled)
- 1 cup cooked chopped spinach
- 1 baked sweet potato (seasoned with a sugar substitute, cinnamon, and vanilla)

Combine this menu with a good, solid workout routine like the one described earlier in this book and you'll be feeling the improved effects in no time. Results can easily yield weight losses of one to two pounds per week. There are fat-free butter substitutes available for cooking, as well as fat-free no-stick sprays for grilling meats. Lemon pepper, sodium-free season-all, cayenne, fresh onion/garlic/bell pepper, cinnamon, sugar substitutes, nutmeg, and allspice help to add flavor to your foods without adding fat and calories.

Remember, ladies, you eat to live, not live to eat! Many adults can take a healthy lesson in eating from children. They don't eat according to a clock, but rather when their bodies tell them they are hungry. They also eat only until they are full, and not necessarily when the bottle, or plate, is empty. This often results in their eating four to eight small meals or snacks a day. It's a healthier method that keeps the body's metabolism working nonstop throughout the day, rather than stopping between meals or trying to overcompensate when the body feels deprived or starved, as with many diets. The key to weight loss and good weight maintenance is to be mindful of what goes into your mouth. Make sure your body is breaking it down and digesting it all day. Good nutrition becomes a lifestyle change, and not a temporary diet followed until a desired weight is reached. The change allows you not only to reach, but to also maintain, the goal you've set.

Now, before you get a long face and think this means no more dinner rolls, cheesecake, and cocktails, let's get one thing straight: if you do choose to indulge in those favorites, it simply means you may need to step up your game a bit more in the fitness portion of your program. These items should not be part of your everyday menu, but rather a weekly, monthly, or special treat that will not have huge negative impacts on your road to optimum nutrition, health, and fitness. To help avoid those temptations, don't keep them in the house. That way, when you get the urge for a snack, you'll be reaching for something healthy instead.

Again, good nutrition doesn't have to be boring. When shared with a partner, it can be fun and flirty and lead to the sweetest lovemaking. Think of it as eating your way to the bedroom! Want to get in the mood with food? Try snacking on bananas and sugar-free popsicles; these can be definite turn-ons for your partner when you do it in a playful, sexual manner. Catch him watching you snack, and turn it into a pleasing tease that lets him know you can do those things to more than just a banana! Set up a nude dessert buffet for your partner one afternoon. Adorn your nude or lingerie-clad body with lots of luscious fresh-cut fruits, strategically laid on all parts of your beautiful body, and allow him to suck, lick, and eat to his heart's content—feeding you a few bites in between so you both can enjoy the tantalizing flavors and aromas emitted by the fruit and each other. Finish it off with spicy, sweet, playful sex! No doubt, next time you're at the grocery store, you'll find yourself reaching for berries and pineapples instead of a bag of cookies or chips!! For an added twist of anticipation, use a blindfold and tease him as you feed him—gently gliding sweet, wet strawberries across his lips, or dripping pineapple juice onto his stomach before you hungrily lick it off and then kiss him with your own tasty, sticky lips. Keep him wondering what you're going to do next.

If that's a bit over the top for you, start slow. Try feeding each other a few berries or cut fruit, teasing the lips before allowing the bite, and taking time to slowly lick each other's fingers while gazing into each other's eyes. If you're indulging in a glass of wine or champagne, slowly undress yourself and your partner and drip small amounts of wine onto his body while allowing him to do the same to yours. Slowly lick the wine from each other's bodies, and see what happens next. The end result will be hot, steamy, sex, and you'll be making healthy, nutritious choices at the same time.

Erotic Info: Your lips are one hundred times more sensitive than the tips of the fingers, and they are even more sensitive than your private areas, which explains why kissing is such a turn-on!

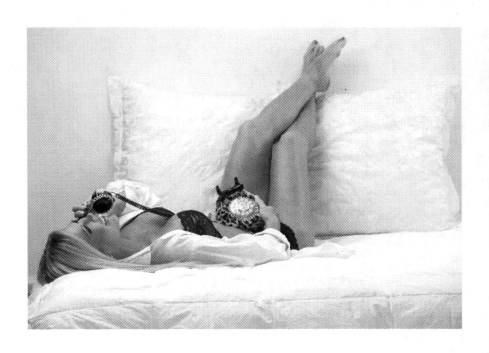

Seduction isn't making someone do what they don't want to do. Seduction is enticing someone into doing what they secretly want to do already.

Walter Rant

~~~~~

Tantalizing Talk, In and Out of the Bedroom

Admit it! We all enjoy getting compliments now and then. One of the greatest gifts you can give or receive is a heartfelt compliment! As much as a woman likes to hear how beautiful and amazing she looks, men also like to know that they are pleasing to their partner physically and sexually. Likes and dislikes in a relationship should be discussed openly, gently, and fairly, and not just those pertaining to the bedroom and sexual relations. Keeping open communication with your partner helps to develop a daily bond and trust that benefits all areas of a relationship. If you can't trust your mate with financial matters, business matters, matters of the household, family matters, and more, you certainly won't be able to trust him with your innermost sexual fears and fantasies. Selfishness has no part in a healthy relationship. By serving your partner, staying tuned in to what he thinks and needs, and building him up, you create an environment that allows him to do the same for you and in the end, you both win.

When you are ready to take that intimate step, a few ground rules should be set *before* you enter the bedroom. If there are certain things that make you uncomfortable or that you absolutely cannot do, it's important to share this with your partner ahead of time so there are no surprises in the bedroom. The heat of the moment is not the best time for him to discover that he's doing something to hurt you physically or emotionally. Share ahead of time so your partner knows how to approach you and how to please you while continuing to gain your trust and show you how much you are loved. If you're afraid or embarrassed to tell him what you don't like, then put a great deal of emphasis on what you *do* like so he will focus on doing those things instead of trying something else. Next, show your partner with your words, actions, and reactions how much you like what is being done! This will ensure that he keeps doing it the way you like it. It takes two to tango in the dance you are creating together, so always remember to return the favor by taking time to learn your partner's likes and dislikes as well. Before you try something new that might be a bit "unusual," discuss it with your partner. When it comes to the bedroom and lovemaking, nothing is off-limits as long as both partners are comfortable with it, it's legal, nobody gets physically or emotionally hurt, and it doesn't involve dragging toxic baggage (or people) into the relationship.

Understanding how the opposite sex thinks plays a big part in how partners respond and react in a relationship. The ultimate goal of sex for a man is the climax and to feel like he satisfied his partner. For a woman, it's the emotional release—climax isn't always necessary for a woman to feel satisfied with the encounter. Men often confuse emotions with sex. They think that the more they have sex with their partner, the more it shows how much they love her. If the partner doesn't respond in kind, the man may feel disconnected and conclude that his partner doesn't love him or want him anymore.

Partners need to understand each other's sexual needs to make sure they are not sending the wrong signals to each other. Sex should not feel like one more chore you are expected to do each day, nor should you be penalized or made to feel insignificant if you don't want to take it to that level every day. Factors like kids, family, jobs, and responsibilities change as a relationship grows and matures, so it's important to continue having discussions about your sex life and what is or isn't working to make sure it stays strong. You can't continue to do the same thing, the same way, with the same frequency, if things around you are constantly changing. Be flexible and reasonable, and communicate constantly with your partner. Just as your needs and desires may change, be understanding of the fact that your partner's may change as well. Understand that men need to be respected, admired, and physically needed. Women, on the other hand, want love, time, and the feeling of being emotionally needed.

Communication is more than just "talking" to each other. We also have to learn to listen carefully and risk being open with each other. It's important that the message being sent is the same as the message being heard. Authentic communication through verbal and nonverbal methods is essential to building intimacy in a relationship. When he talks to you, listen intently. Stay in the moment, keep eye contact, nod, and be willing to ask a question or two to show you're trying to understand where he's coming from.

Body language and posture speak volumes, so be careful what your body is saying. Crossed arms and having your body turned away from him may send the message that you don't want to be bothered. Face him instead. If you're sitting, even part your legs a bit to let him know you're "open" to whatever he's got on his mind. Let him know you're turned on by touching his inner thigh, or caressing the nape of his neck or arm as you're talking, but make sure your eye contact and focus are still on him and the conversation. Don't get too distracted by his sexy, strong arms or tight muscles. If he's naked or wearing shorts, stroking the inner thigh works well, not only because it's so close to his genitals, but also because it's a sensitive area with lots of nerve endings. The inner thigh also is more tender than the rest of the muscle-bound thigh.

Men love to see us smile, as long as it's sincere. Depending on the conversation, you should decide whether your smile should be shy and coy, or big and flirty. If he's trying to say something serious or talk to you about his insecurities, you certainly don't want to be sitting there grinning like a Cheshire cat. However, if he's talking fantasies and letting you know what he wants to do to you later, a big smile is just the invitation he needs to let him know that you are just as excited.

To spice up your communication, every so often pick a sexy topic to discuss while you're finishing up dinner, or getting ready for bed. Talk about your fantasies, something you've read, or something you've seen in a movie or on TV that you might like to try. Ever wonder why so many women read romance novels? Simple. They love romance!! They love to fantasize that they are the lead character being seduced. Why leave it between the covers of a book when you can bring it between the sheets in your own bedroom? Share your fantasies with your partner, either in conversation or by reading him a few pages of the novel you're reading. Ask your partner if he likes it when you talk dirty during sex, or how he feels when you touch yourself. This might seem silly, but if you start talking dirty in a manner that makes your partner wonder who you really are, it could have an adverse effect. Touching yourself a certain way might make him wonder if he's needed at all in the bedroom, or he might feel that you're taking that pleasure of touch away from him. Everyone acts and reacts differently, so communicate!!

Men like:

- Watching you put on your high heels.

- Reading and rereading the sweet, sexy texts and e-mails they receive from you during the day.

- Being complimented on their bodies. Men are sometimes more insecure about their bodies than we realize.

- You to try new things—food, hairstyles, fantasies, clothes …

- Seeing you in their button-down dress shirts or oversized T-shirts, or walking around the house in comfortable clothes with no bra underneath.

- To get dressed and strut their stuff as you watch.

- To be spooned really hard and deep off and on, all night long.

- To watch you taking a bubble bath, especially if you have "bath toys" and invite them to join.

- To watch you working out good and hard, sweating and panting.

- To watch you being playful with your girlfriends—laughing, talking, dancing.

- For you to send them a self-made videotape or phone video—it doesn't have to be X-rated either.

- For you to be comfortable touching yourself.

- To receive special notes or sex-texts during the day letting them know they're special and reminding them about the previous hot night or what's to come later.

- To be surprised when they come to bed. They shouldn't always know what's going to happen!

- The list is endless!! Talk to your man, and fill in the rest of the blanks together!!

Remember, when you're communicating, what you say is as

important as what you don't say. How you touch him can make him pull you in closer or get up and walk away. Let your passion shine. Be open and look enthusiastic. Laugh out loud, speak confidently, and be kind and sweet toward him. Make him your focus, and aim to serve and please him. He'll feel like a king, and will in turn treat you like his queen! Allow yourself a little extra time on occasions when you're getting ready for a night out on the town. This is a perfect opportunity to be spontaneous when you're looking good and smelling good—let him get that "quickie" before you leave; it'll give him something to think about all evening!

Ladies, here are a few more sex secrets we'll share with you before moving along:

- Blindfolds are fun and not only build trust but also force you to rely on senses other than your sight. They can heighten your experience tremendously!

- Touch each other, and not just in the bedroom. Hold his hand. Squeeze his arm. Stroke his fingers. When you pass him in the kitchen, give him a firm squeeze on the butt or other parts of the body, or slide your hand softly along his back as you walk by.

- Sex-text him during the day! Send him a text message when he's at work or least expects to receive it. The message can be sexy, playful, or just a sincere line to let him know that he's all you've been thinking about all day.

- Be spontaneous. When he's watching television and you walk by, flip your shirt up and give him a quick peep show, but keep on walking. Next time you're in an elevator alone, grab him and kiss him hard. The element of surprise is surprisingly stimulating and passionate.

Flirty Fact: Outside of the bedroom, the most common place for adults in the United States to have sex is in the car.

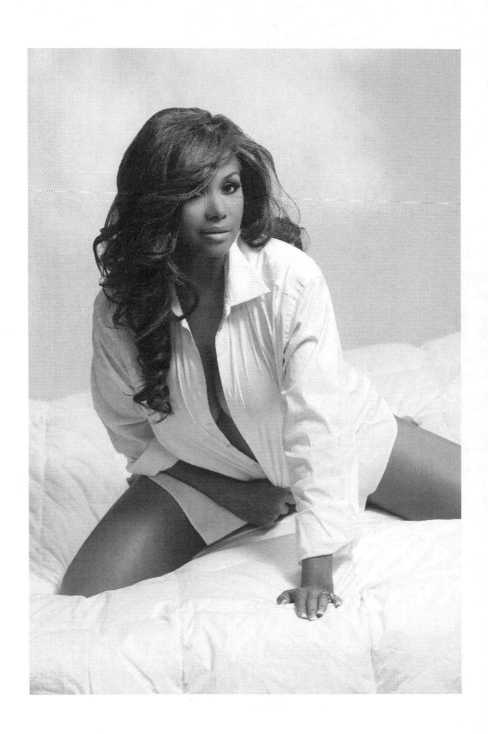

Love is something that never goes out of style.

Beyonce

Chapter Five

Getting Ready for That "Good Good"

We can't help but think that if every woman put as much time into her relationship as she does her job, her children, and her business, those relationships would be awesome! During the weeks before a pageant, we put a lot of time and effort into managing our diets, selecting the right clothes, and tending to our hair/nails/skin to make sure they're flawless. We practice how we should talk, how we should walk, and how we should present ourselves. We fuss over even the smallest details to make sure everything is in order for a perfect presentation. So why not do that when you're getting ready for that "good good"? Each day, you should be aware of your diet, hair, skin, and nails. Choose outfits—whether for work, play, or the bedroom—that show off your best assets and are eye-catching and appealing.

"I'm saving 'it' for just the right time." Here we go again, making excuses. "It" can be anything from that sexy new lingerie to a new hairstyle to a new position you want to try. Don't wait until it's "the right time" … be sexy *now*!!! Oftentimes, women put things off until we think it's time to be romantic or intimate, saving our "best" for the perfect moment—our best makeup, our best hair, our best outfit. Why wait? Why put off being sexy to tomorrow when we can do it right now? To put off until later is to indicate that "now" is not important enough. If you think your partner won't appreciate your sexy lingerie until you lose more weight, you're sadly mistaken. If you think your partner won't like seeing you dolled up in the middle of the day, in the middle of the week, guess again! Remember that communication and how you present yourself to your partner play key roles in the success of your relationship.

Our excuses will talk us right out of a sexy situation every time! It's the same as saving your good china or best clothes for later. You save it for so long, that it eventually goes out of style or no longer fits, and you're ready for something new before you've ever enjoyed what you already have. So what if it's Tuesday afternoon? Put on that hot new nightie with your "too high to walk too far" stiletto heels, and meet him at the front door when he gets home. Better yet, toss your coat/jacket over it, and pick him up at the office. So what if it seems "kinky"; if he likes it, then it's okay. Stop trying to reason about what is right and wrong in a healthy relationship. Bring sexy back! Go out and get it, and stop waiting for it to creep back in on its own at some predestined "right time." If it feels right to you, and right to your partner, then apparently it's the right time, right now! Sexy is a state of mind, so free yourself and free your mind to do what is pleasing to your partner and you. Unveil the hidden fantasies—his and yours!

Speaking of unveiling, try unleashing some new hairdos and see what happens. Wigs, weaves, and extensions can quickly become "helpers" in your relationship because they can allow playful changes without compromising your real locks if you're not yet ready for a drastic permanent change. Your partner may be turned on by white lace lingerie and long, straight hair. Perhaps he fantasizes about a woman in a red bodice trimmed with black, and short, spiked, edgy hair to match. Whatever the mood, you can change and spice it up with a few highlights or extensions without damaging your natural hair. Wigs are great because you have the flexibility to change color, length, texture, and style in a matter of minutes. A sex kitten one minute can change into a boardroom executive the next, or become a blond bombshell in just minutes—literally. They're also great for spontaneous events when you don't have time to get your hair done or washed and set. If your partner's dropping by in fifteen minutes, you can shower, shave, and lotion down in twelve, and secure a great wig in three, and look like a million bucks when he arrives at the door.

Extensions, too, are a great way to gain length and thickness. They can offer excellent highlights, and no one needs to know it's not your real hair except for your stylist and you. Try them out, and if you don't like them, have them removed. It's simple as that. Believe us, most women are wearing them!

Whether you choose wigs, extensions, or your own natural hair, make sure it's "bedroom" hair. That simply means make sure it's clean, smells good, and feels good to the touch. Make it an extension of your body, and an asset to your sexiness. A man is stimulated by the sense of touch, and he enjoys touching your face, your skin, your hair, and your whole body! If you're self-conscious about his running his fingers through your extension or wig, then by all means, try something else. You don't want to send the wrong signal and make him think his touch is what's making you nervous. Whatever you wear, whatever you do, whatever role you play should be fun and comfortable and allow you to release your inhibitions, not hide behind them.

Hair isn't the only thing you should pay special attention to on a regular basis. Makeup can also play its part in bringing out your sensuality and beauty. Try different makeup styles to see what your partner does and does not respond to. When your natural beauty shines through, there's a tendency to think that no makeup is needed. This might be right, but even the most beautiful women can enhance their glow, even if it's only with a little bit of mascara and blush, or a hint of lipstick or gloss.

A woman's moods, menstrual cycle, hormones, and more can play tricks on her complexion from time to time, so don't get stuck in a rut of always or never wearing makeup. Be attuned to your skin each day. You know what works best for you, and you know what makes you feel sexiest. If your partner likes you all "glammed up" from head to toe, then don't be surprised if when you come in with rollers, no makeup, a cotton nightgown, and fuzzy slippers, he rolls over and goes to sleep. If that's how he's used to seeing you all the time and he still gets excited and turned on, then imagine how much more enticed he'll be to see you periodically donned in something silky and lacy, with long, soft locks, smelling like you just stepped out of a shower of the best fragrance he's ever smelled. You thought the sex was hot before!!?? Try it now!!! While women are stimulated emotionally from within, men are excited by touch, smell, and sight. So let your partner see you at your best. Let him see you sexy. Let him see you confident. Let him see you "nude"—unveiled, uncovered, and unleashed, and ready to love him.

It comes down to learning about your partner and the small things that make a difference to him. Be intriguing, spontaneous, and fun. Present to him a partner who is confident and sexy, and finger-licking good! Make him want it … need it … crave it! When he knows you've got that "good good" waiting for him at home, and that you love and trust him, he'll be beating down the door to get home every night!!

Naughty Notation: Although nearly any body part or item of clothing may be an object of sexual fetish, the shoe and the foot are the two most common fetishes in the Western society.

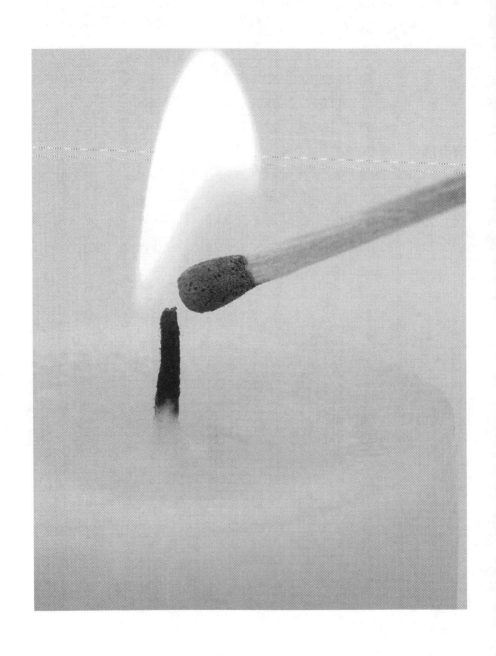

In a great romance, each person basically plays a part that the other really likes.

Elizabeth Ashley

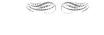

Chapter Six

Let the Bedroom Games Begin

A man falls in love with a woman because of how she makes him feel about himself. Make him feel like the king of his castle, the head of his household, like a million bucks, and he's not going anywhere. Want to really boost his ego? Then let him know when he does something pleasurable to you. Heavy moans and groans, deep "aahhhhs" and "oohhhhs" let him know when it's "just right." Soft whispers of "Don't stop … yessss … Lick me there …" all let him know that he's satisfying you immensely. He loves the control he feels by making you lose yourself in him when making love. When you've got him on cloud nine, totally into pleasing you and completely attuned to what you are sharing with him, take advantage of the moment and remind him of your fantasies.

Gaining trust in the bedroom goes a long way, as does gaining trust in the relationship. Sometimes the pressures of life can cause us to neglect passion and playfulness in our relationships. All couples need to energize and nurture their passion toward each other to keep the relationship going and growing. There are playful bedroom games you can play together that build intimacy and break down insecurities so that you can build trust.

Hide-and-seek was fun when we were children because there was a sense of anticipation as you hunted for the others. The same is true in your sex life. How exciting and enticing to have a trail of clothing welcoming your partner home in the evening. He's greeted at the door by a pair of blue jeans that you've stepped out of, and a little further he sees the shirt you've maneuvered out of. He rounds the corner to see the bra you've slipped off and let fall to the floor, and the panties a few feet further. He's already visualizing what lies ahead! The anticipation of what he will find makes him eager to play a flirty game of "you're it!" Want to be a bit more seductive? A trail of candles or rose petals can also lead the way to the treasure that is waiting for him behind closed doors.

Show-and-tell is another great game we all learned as children and can incorporate into the bedroom. Show him yours, and he'll show you his. Show him what you like, and tell him how you'd like him to do it to you! Perhaps you tell him to undress you, item by item. Maybe you show him different body parts and tell him which ones to kiss, lick, squeeze, pinch, or suck. The ideas for this one are endless. Just use your imagination!

Body massage is also a great way to relax and please each other through sensual touch. Massage creates a period of bonding that can bring back laughter and amusement. It allows you to tap in to your inner self to bring out positive energy to share with one another. The right touch is often more powerful and seductive than a word or even a kiss. Always remember that sensual body massage is not a selfish act for your own pleasure, but rather an expression of your desire to please your partner. When your partner is pleased, you will be too! Here are a few things to help entice all of your body senses during a massage:

- Scented candles
- Creamy, warm lotions or massage oils
- Soft, gentle lighting, perhaps even in different colors
- Silky sheets and pillows that you can slip, slide, and roll on
- Your favorite sexy, sensual music
- Hot bubble bath or a steamy shower for two (For those of you who are a bit more daring, consider gently shaving each other's genital areas. Not quite that risqué? Then just stick to lathering each other all over, slowly and gently!)
- Privacy, patience, and an open mind to help set the mood
- And, of course, your "Pillow Talk" Pillow!

While we're on the subject of body massage, bubble baths, and shaving, here's a hot new topic to consider—"manscaping"! Yes, that's right, we said "manscaping." The art of manscaping means to groom a man in his private, personal areas as a way to reduce odors and discomfort and increasing hygiene and overall appeal to his partner. Body grooming is no longer just a feminine fancy. When it comes to grooming, it's not about being masculine or feminine; it's about being trimmed, neat, and clean. Most men will not be as open to trimming and shaving as women are, but in certain places, it's definitely better off than on!

The first thing to remember in the art of manscaping is to simply take away the stigma associated with masculine body hair removal. If you are just getting used to the idea of shaving or removing your own genital hair, remember to be open to the idea that men actually might want to try it too. It really does enhance your body. It provides easy access to those sensual areas, feels wonderful to the touch, is visually pleasing to the eye, and makes the area much easier to keep clean and reduce odors. You don't have to feel embarrassed or awkward for taking it all off; it's a very freeing feeling, and more women—and men—are doing it than you probably imagine.

Body grooming is something that you and your partner can do together. Try different ways that are comfortable for each of you. Electric razors work great for men, who may not want the same clean closeness that most women desire from a wax or shave. When considering manscaping, let's start from the top and work our way down. And remember to use plenty of moisturizer after grooming each area to prevent razor burn or irritation. Important upper areas for a man to consider grooming are his eyebrows (especially if they've grown into a "unibrow"), his shoulders, his back, and his armpits (though this area usually is not groomed down as much as some of the others, but just enough to appear neat and help reduce odor). Eyebrows can be treated quickly with simple tweezing. You don't want them to appear too manicured, as with waxing. You want to keep them looking natural, but neat. Waxing works great on backs and shoulders, and even chests, if you want that finished look and smooth feel. Removing chest hair allows a better visual of a man's muscular structure, especially if he works out regularly and has a nice, even tan. Removing upper body hair lets a man feel cooler, cleaner, and fresher.

Genital grooming also has its advantages. In addition to visually enhancing his "package" by eliminating the surrounding distractions, it reduces odor and moisture retention that might lead to irritation. Oral sex is much more pleasant for both men and women when they're not trying to move hair out of the way all the time. Men with a hairy bottom might want to try trimming it or actually having it removed via laser treatment to prevent it from growing back. It's all a matter of preference for each man and his partner. Don't forget that most men also need to pay attention to trimming and grooming nose and ear hair, too, when necessary. It's okay to remind a man to tackle the back of his neck when getting regular haircuts. After all, one of the first things a woman likes to do when she gets close to a man is caress the nape of his neck. She might be trying to excite him, or she might be checking his grooming techniques—so, men, make sure you're on top of your game!

Manscaping and body grooming can be as personal or as romantic as you want to make it; just make sure you get it done whether you do it yourself or with your partner. Sharing a glass of wine while soft music plays in the background helps to enhance the task and allow it to become a form of foreplay rather than just another routine task. It's a great way to bond in the bedroom. If you're not fully comfortable doing it together, then try leaving the bathroom door slightly ajar so you can watch each other. It's always fun to see your partner preparing his body for what's to come! Oh, and one more little note for those of you starting to notice a few gray hairs popping up in unexpected places—you can purchase nonirritating hair color designed for intimate use that comes in a variety of colors, from black to brown to blond, and everything in between.

Here are some more of our sensual suggestions to add some intrigue to an otherwise stagnant routine:

- How about simply changing your bedroom by just moving furnishings, adding beautiful, soft, silk-covered bedding or pillows, or adding seductive lighting and music to give the feel of a more exotic environment.

- Try a dusting of perfume on your sheets and pillows to inspire a mood and create an aroma of romance each day, so he remembers all day long the sweet smell of the bed that you two share together.

- Leave a little something behind in the bed with your scent on it. Bet he'll have his nose buried in it throughout the day while he's thinking about what he's going to do with you, or to you, the next time he sees you.

- Add fresh flowers and love notes all around the

bedroom and bathroom where the two of you indulge yourselves in each other.

- Do you ever sleep nude? If it's something you don't usually do, give it a try.

- Turn off the television, and turn on the music with your favorite slow jams or playlist.

- Write a love note on the bathroom mirror in red lipstick letting him know you've been thinking about him all day and all night.

- Have you ever bought a pair of furry high-heeled slippers and worn them to bed? Better yet, keep them on after you get into the bed while you're having sex! Try it, and see how he likes it!

- Walk into the room and ask him if he likes your brand-new stiletto heels, and make sure you're wearing nothing else but the shoes.

- We suggest using low-watt red lightbulbs in a couple of lamps in the bedroom. This will add a beautiful, soft sunset effect to the room and a sexy glimmer on your naked body.

- Set a pallet of soft pillows on the floor and make love to him there instead of in the bed.

- Ladies, you must remember that keeping the atmosphere sexy and seductive is a must. Use your fireplace, lights, music, scents, and more to entice your partner. Become his goddess of love, the one he will remember and love, forever.

Whatever you choose, just remember that bedroom games don't have to be long, elaborate role-playing events, unless that's what you like. Short, sweet, spontaneous "quickies" can be just as fun. A few minor changes can easily entice and enhance the mood and let him know you're ready to play. Men love the game of seduction even if you've been dating for a while or are married. When you keep the proverbial ball rolling, it continues to get bigger and better, always changing shape and style to keep the relationship revived and stimulated. Don't forget to love red in the bed! By that, we mean pull out your red dress, your red lingerie, your red stilettos, and red lipstick! Make it red hot!!! Make sure you have a comfortable temperature in the room where you are making love. Extremely cold temperatures can make it more difficult to reach climax. Of course, that also may mean that you just have to find some new ways to warm things up!

As with most games, sex and lovemaking goes more smoothly when it is able to flow uninterrupted. Why risk breaking the mood because you're digging through a bedside drawer for your toys and lotions? The fear of having someone discover these intimate items often leads us to hide them in the back of the bottom nightstand drawer, in a box under the bed, or between the mattress and box spring. How unromantic is it to leave your partner's warm embrace so you can crawl under the bed for your "stuff"? A simple idea is to have a special bag or hideaway pillow that stays on the bed but is designed in such a manner that it complements the bedding and décor and remains undetected and unidentifiable to anyone else who may come into your room throughout the day. The Nude "Pillow Talk" Pillow is a perfect solution and is available in different colors and styles to complement your bedroom style. Once you get started, there's now no reason to stop until you're both thoroughly satisfied.

A simple suggestion to keep in mind is that foreplay is not something that should happen after you get into bed and are ready to have sex. It should begin the minute you awake, each and every day. Even if you're not sure if you're going to have sex that night, your partner should know that you want him and that you are thinking and preparing for that special time, whenever it does happen to occur. Long glances while getting dressed or preparing meals, flirtatious e-mails or texts, love notes intimately placed in briefcases or lunch kits, a hot, steamy kiss as you leave for work—all of these things help to stimulate your partner and remind him that you've got something special waiting for him later on. It takes commitment and effort to stay in sync with each other. Both partners have to want it, and both partners have to show it, continually, not just during sex.

Ladies, definitely don't forget the "after-play"! Just as foreplay is so important to getting in the mood, after-play is just as important to remind each other how good it was. How you respond after can affect how your partner responds next time. For a woman, the tenderness and affection after lovemaking seal the deal and remind her that she satisfies her partner. When a partner jumps up immediately to take a shower or check a cell phone, it sends a message that the other partner is no longer needed. If you don't discuss and share with your partner how you feel after sex, a wall can develop, and insecurities can begin to mount that will prevent your being able to unleash and unveil your inner sensuality later on in the relationship.

Arousing Aphrodisiac: The average person spends two whole weeks of their life kissing … that's an average of 336 hours. (This is an average we'd personally like to try and beat!)

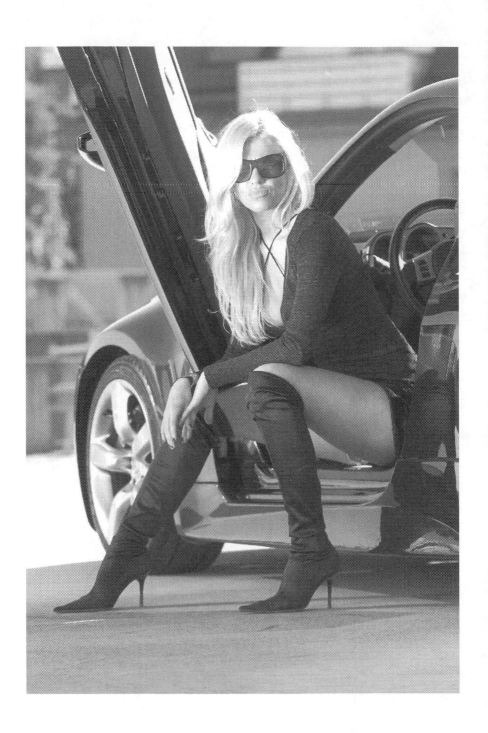

By having the courage to be yourself, you put something wonderful in the world that was not there before.

Edwin Elliot

⚭ ⚭

Chapter Seven

Revving Up for Round Two

Too often we get caught up in our daily routines and treat lovemaking as though it's just another task that needs to be completed. How often do we complete the act, wash off, and then simply get ready for bed? As young adults, we found time and ways to sometimes stay in bed together for hours, trying to achieve multiple orgasms—so caught up in the heat of the moment that we never wanted it to end. As careers, housework, kids, and daily chores crept in, the time for sex and lovemaking became less and less, and we wonder why our sex lives seem stagnant at times. As we mature, it's important that we still strive for those sexual marathons that bring climax and release again and again, to reassure ourselves and our partners that we are satisfied and secure in the relationship.

Men don't fall in love with one certain body part; they fall in love with the complete package. A woman who is totally comfortable with herself and every inch of her body can reveal her true essence to her partner. Know yourself, love yourself, and be yourself. Some partners enjoy the inclusion of "toys" in their sexual relationship. However, make sure this is part of your communication before you get intimate in order to avoid any embarrassing or sudden surprises. Some women do not like the idea of using vibrators or toys. For others, those good vibrations keep their sex lives charged up. It's important to remember, though, that since your partner is involved, your actions should ultimately be to please and not exclude him. Vibrators and masturbation may physically stimulate you while also visually stimulating your partner. But make sure your partner is involved in the moment of release to avoid making him feel disconnected or deprived of a pleasure that belonged to him. Allow your partner to help you hold and move the vibrator, or show him how you like it done. Ladies, try using a small vibrator against your cheek when pleasuring your partner orally—the added vibrations will provide new and unusual sensations for him. Another trick to enhancing oral sex is to dissolve a small menthol cough drop in your mouth prior to taking him orally. It can cause a very pleasing sensation for him. Make it lemon flavored to avoid smelling too much like a hospital ward in the bedroom—there's nothing sexy about that! Ladies, one more tip to remember is that men like to have some parts of their genitals licked, kissed, and sucked gently and carefully!! This adds pleasure and wonderful stimulation for him.

By the way, who says sex has to happen only in the bedroom? Or for that matter, only indoors? Outdoor sex can be exciting and fun, and provides a sense of adventure that you won't find indoors!

Balconies, plush lawns adorned in soft blankets, hammocks, and lawn furniture all provide great outlets for outdoor lovemaking. Whether it's during an early-morning sunrise, a quiet springtime afternoon while the kids are all at school, or a romantic evening under the stars, just make sure your outdoor area offers privacy and seclusion—you certainly don't want the neighbors sharing in your afternoon delight from their upstairs windows. Is your husband a hunter, fisherman, or outdoorsman? Sex in the woods under a big, shady tree, or on the bank of a secluded lake or stream can be awesome, but make sure to take precautions against mosquitoes and other outside critters. The next time you have to park in a parking garage at a mall, office, or event, try a spontaneous quickie in the backseat! Double-check first for security cameras; you certainly don't want to find yourself in an embarrassing position! The same is true for those of you who've ever considered a little dressing-room dare. Make sure it's mostly private with no two-way mirrors. If the coast is clear (and you're not being electronically monitored), let your partner help you get into, and especially out of, a few outfits. He may want to let his hands linger in certain places, or he may want you to try on something else for fit, if you catch our drift!!!

Turn your Mile High Club fantasy into a reality. Talk and flirt about it the next time you fly, and get your creative juices flowing. Let your man know you're going to take him for a mind-blowing ride as soon as you reach your destination. The next time you're at the movies, sit in the back and make out like you did when you were teenagers. Hold hands, feed each other popcorn, kiss, touch, laugh, and just experience the thrill of new love all over again. Have you ever made out on an airplane, in a limousine, in a hot tub, or on a cruise ship? Try it!

One of the most sensual and romantic experiences that we shared with our husbands is our venture to Bellagio while on vacation. One afternoon, we took a private excursion on a beautifully crafted sailboat from Lake Como to Bellagio (which is considered by some to be the most beautiful town in all of Europe). The entire scene was a picturesque combination of tranquil, peaceful, made-to-order weather along with a glorious landscape of rolling, adventurous mountains on either side of the lake. It was a breathtaking atmosphere unmatched by anything we'd seen before. As we sailed past enchanting celebrity villas, we laughed and talked and shared stories with our husbands of romantic escapades and ideas of how sexy and exciting it would be to have an opportunity to make love in a sailboat on a day such as the one we were experiencing. What an unforgettable adventure that would be!

If going completely outdoors is just a bit over the top for you, experiment with other rooms in the house and even the garage. Steal back that excitement you got necking in the backseat of the car when you were teenagers. Get creative in the kitchen or bathroom. Rediscover where you live, and try something new on the kitchen counters, in the backyard pool, or on the hood of your car. Even a clean, oversized, neatly kept closet holds a certain intrigue. Our favorite thing to do when we buy a new home, or rent a place for vacation, is to "christen" every room with some sort of sexual activity, including bathrooms, closets, and laundry rooms! If you have a home office, act out one of those office scenes like you've seen on television. Sweep the desktop contents onto the floor and engage in your own private office party right there on top of the desk.

Most couples are familiar with foreplay, leading up to sex,

and even with the term *after-play*, which refers to the act of intimacy and romance immediately following sex. But what about "mid-play?" That's just a term we coined meaning to continue caressing, sharing, and playing in between the climaxes. If you're lucky enough to carve out more than an hour together, it's much easier to stay in bed and talk and play between multiple acts of intercourse. Don't let your busy lifestyle stop you, though, from enjoying multiple orgasms in a single day. There's no rule that says because you had sex in the morning, you can't have it again until the next day. The excitement that comes with multiple orgasms is greatly increased when there is continual activity and mid-play taking place between releases. Mid-play says, "That was great, but I'm not done with you yet!!" There might be time for a quickie in the morning; but don't let it end there.

After you each start into your daily routine, try these forms of mid-play to keep it hot until the next encounter, which could come as soon as mid-morning, lunchtime, or before dinner. Don't wait until the next day if the opportunity presents itself sooner. These are a few naughty tricks that work for us:

- Be creative with a sex-text—send a picture of just a body part (breasts, lips, hands). I once sent my husband a picture of my beautiful foot after a pedicure and reminded him that it would soon be sliding its way up the back of his thighs.

- When you pass in the hallway, expose yourself quickly and teasingly; raise your shirt, playfully squeeze your breasts, suck your index finger.

- At the breakfast table, choose a banana for a

quick snack and play with it a little bit while he's watching.

- Put a piece of underwear or lingerie on the seat of his car so he'll remember to hurry back from wherever he's going.

The ideas for mid-play are endless, and it's a great opportunity to have fun and tease each other despite busy lifestyles. Whether you find opportunity for three, four, or even five quickies in the same day, or get lucky enough to steal away for a two-hour marathon at a nearby hotel, take advantage of every sexual opportunity you have together. It will make those long, drawn-out, separated days less lonely, because you'll know what's to come.

Remember, the key here is finding the *you* in every new sexual adventure. Build a bridge between who *you* are at your core and a new sexual experience that lies a few feet outside of the person you have defined yourself to be. "The creation of something new is not accomplished by the intellect but by the play instinct acting from inner necessity. The creative mind plays with the objects it loves" (Carl Jung, Swiss psychiatrist, influential thinker, and the founder of analytical psychology).

Teasing Tidbit: Headaches may be cured by having intercourse. Research indicates that powerful endorphins and painkillers are released during orgasm.

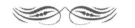

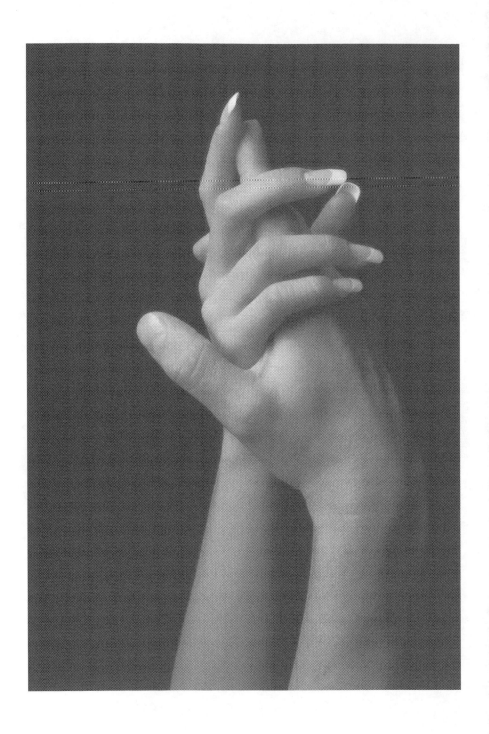

The most important ingredient you put into any relationship is not what you say or what you do, but what and who you are.

Stephen R. Covey

≈≈

Chapter 8

Recipe for a Yummy Sexual Relationship

Think about your favorite recipe and the special, tantalizing ingredients that combine together to make it so delectable. The mix of flavors, aromas, and textures leads to an entree that delights and satisfies all the senses of your body. What is it that makes *you* love your favorite meal? Is it the way it looks, the way its tastes, or how it smells? Whatever it is that delights your taste buds when you're eating your favorite food, the same is true for great sex! It takes the right mix of sensual, pleasurable ingredients to delight and satisfy all your senses. The recipe includes ingredients that stimulate you emotionally, intellectually, intimately, and physically. Of course, nothing can replace the tried and true recipe of a heaping of beauty inside and out. However, let's talk about a few additional ingredients to keep in the mix for a healthy, pleasing sexual relationship:

- We agree that friendship and trust are two of the most important.

- Frequent, yummy, playful sex (but someone has to initiate it).

- Being emotionally thoughtful and demonstrating your feelings.

- Here's another of our favorites—spontaneous sex (this includes orally) … anytime, anywhere, and often.

- Uplifting conversation (Would you believe that some couples don't know how to talk to each other when they're alone?)

- This one's a winner—de-stressing! You have to learn to let go of the stress so you don't carry it into the bedroom with you. Sometimes, you don't even realize the stress you're under until you finally let it go.

- One-on-one time at home, during social events, and on vacations.

- Keep dating, no matter how long you've been together or been married. We have date night every Friday; it's a critical part of our week, just like going to work.

- Remain sexy (Need we stress the importance of this one?!)

- Give respect, and get respect. Compliments go a long way, and there's no such thing as "too many."

- Communicate—talk it out, whatever it is. Mutual

communication can be so therapeutic and beneficial to your soul. A good talk is sometimes more satisfying than sex!

- Keep things hot, spicy, and exciting. And remember to add a little humor now and then as well.
- You have to be willing to say "I'm sorry" or "I was wrong" every once in a while
- Remember the little things that are pleasing to your spouse, and repeat them as often as possible.
- Be considerate toward each other, and treat each other the way you'd want to be treated.
- Say "I love you," "I adore you," "I want you," "I think you're hot."

An ounce of respect and large servings of love and honesty can go a very long way in a relationship and lead to an endless plateful of sensual and passionate sex. If really good lovemaking gets you emotional or teary-eyed, don't hold back. Allow your tears of joy to flow freely, and let your man know that he makes you feel that terrific.

Don't be afraid to offer a few leftovers now and then. Too many couples think that lovemaking has to be a drawn-out ritual. Think about a special Sunday dinner that takes hours to prepare. When it's done, you are full, satisfied, and content. Most likely, when Monday rolls around, you're still thinking about the leftovers. You may not want to fully indulge again, but a little taste of something is definitely calling your name. The same holds true for good sex. You take time one evening to bathe each other, to fully massage each other's bodies until the passion is so overwhelming you can't hold back any longer. The silk underwear (his and hers) fall quickly to the floor; hands grope and caress; lips kiss, lick, tease, and suck; bodies mesh together and move rhythmically until they explode into a sweet, sticky dessert of their own. Wow! Once again you are full, satisfied, and content. And just like after the meal, the next day you're still thinking about the sex and wondering what leftovers might be available when you get home. These "leftovers" could be anything from a quickie as soon as you walk in the door to tasty, finger-licking oral sex before bedtime. Whatever it turns out to be, the memory and excitement of the previous night's course are still fresh in your mind, further enhancing the pleasantness of the leftovers. There's no rule that says it always has to be a full course to be satisfying. Learn to indulge in the moment together, no matter how long or how short it may be, and understand that when the leftovers start to run out, it's time to fix up another mind-blowing full-course meal and start the feeding frenzy all over again.

Delectable Detail: Many of the ingredients in chocolate are proven to cause arousal. In fact, some experts believe chocolate may even be more effective than foreplay for creating arousal.

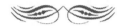

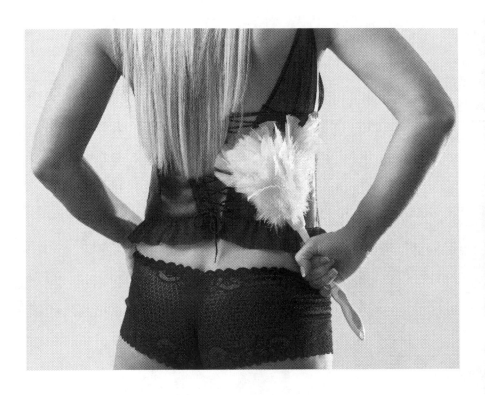

Love is just a word until someone comes along
and gives it meaning.

Unknown

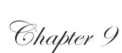

Chapter 9

Spring-Clean Your Sex Life

Just as you spring-clean your home and closets, periodically
you need to spring-clean your sex life to keep it from
getting stale and worn-out. What worked five, fifteen, or
thirty years ago when you entered the relationship may no longer
be the secret to keeping your partner craving more of that "good
good." There are certain things that men and women must do
in order to keep the relationship sexy, hot, and thriving.

Some of the cleaning is easy, like keeping your wardrobe,
hairstyle, and makeup current and appealing. Keep your home
and bedroom clean as well so that you can "sex" your partner
whenever, and wherever, you both feel like it. Not so easy is
making sure you stay on top of changes that might be happening
with your emotions and your physical self. It's not easy when
you're juggling kids, work, household chores, and your partner.

But as women, it's important that we find time to ourselves to be alone in prayer, meditation, reflection—whatever puts you into a totally relaxed, calm state of mind, so that your mind, body, and soul can replenish and revitalize in order to remain refreshed, healthy, positive, and sexy inside and out each and every day. You must take care of *you*—the essence of who you are, your innermost intimacy, your "nudeness" that makes up the total you that we talked about in Chapter One.

Remember to consult your nutritionist or doctor as you mature to make sure hormones stay in balance. You might find it necessary to use lubricants periodically to avoid uncomfortable friction during intercourse. This isn't something to be embarrassed about. Talk to your partner so there are no misunderstandings. A man may think a woman is no longer "excited" by his touch because she doesn't quickly produce the same lubrication as before. Share with him the changes happening in your body so that he can change his techniques if necessary to help you both achieve satisfaction. Shop together for products on the market that aid in sexual lubrication. Natural oral lubrication always gets the job done as well, and it's always available! Not only will this build trust, but it also can be enticing to both of you as you read the labels and advertisements telling about how it will work! Labeling like, "enhance her sexual pleasure," "increased lubrication," or "heightened arousal," is enough to get any man's blood flowing to the right places!

You also need to "spring-clean" your routine. If you and your partner have been doing the same position for ten years, it's time to try something new. If you've been wearing the same style of nightgown or lingerie, spice it up with something different. Change your foreplay, and your after-play, and open up the communication with your partner to find out if he's still turned on by what goes on in your private life. Have his fantasies changed? Have the old ones been fulfilled yet? Is there anything new he'd like to try? Is there anything old he'd like to stop? Oftentimes couples think if it's not broke, why fix it? Instead, they should be thinking, "This works great; how can it be improved!?"

Don't be afraid to do something different in your everyday routine—a long weekend getaway, a night at a fancy hotel, a play or concert that requires you to dress more fancifully than usual, or dinner at a romantic restaurant you've always wanted to visit.

Here are a few more things you can try:

- Call your husband to meet you for drinks or appetizers, and wear something sleek and sexy he's never seen.

- Plan an evening like you did when you first started dating—dinner and a movie, with no expectations afterward. (At some point, some of you might want to go even deeper than that and consider actually renewing your wedding vows.)

- Visit an erotica store together and shop for something you both want to try.

- Attend an event that neither of you has ever been exposed to before, like an opera or symphony.

- Go for a quiet dusk/evening drive down a country road and bring a blanket to lie on under the stars somewhere secluded along the way.

- Chill a bottle of wine, light the fireplace or a few candles, turn off all the other lights in the house, and just sit and talk with your partner about anything and everything that comes to mind—childhood memories, life's favorites, dreams for the future …

- Find out what makes you both happy, and simply do more of it!

Isn't it funny how we can jump up and do a quick cleanup in the house if friends call to say they're on their way over? Just as we are always willing to do a little here and there for friends, remember to also do a little here and there each day for your relationship. Keep the turn-ons and turn-offs at the forefront of your thoughts so that you always can react quickly, spontaneously, and effectively to please your partner. What does he like? Femininity, sexual spontaneity, a healthy partner, good humor, independence and confidence, a kind spirit, ongoing romance and tenderness—your list can go on and on. Those are the things you should make part of the routine each and every day, and night. Stay away from turn-offs like being abrasive and argumentative, being insulting, criticizing, exhibiting poor health and not taking care of yourself, nagging, sloppiness, disinterest, and always being predictable. You've got to mix it up a bit and make the most of the assets that are pleasing to your partner. You know what you excel in at work, how your boss likes it done, and how to execute it. Try the same approach in your relationship!

Stimulating Truth: The vibrator, a common sex toy for women, was originally designed in the nineteenth century as a medication to combat the anxiety-related symptoms of "hysteria" (now known as menstruation).

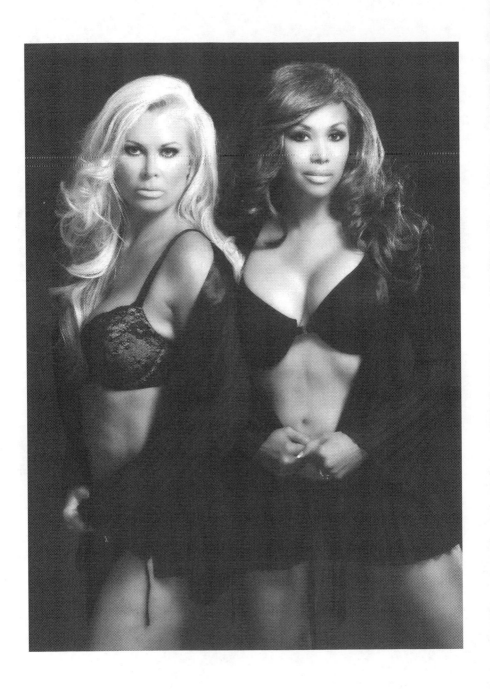

Love is like a friendship caught on fire. In the beginning a flame, very pretty, often hot and fierce, but still only light and flickering. As love grows older, our hearts mature and our love becomes as coals, deep-burning and unquenchable.

Bruce Lee

Chapter 10
Keep It Hot, and Keep It Coming

When it's all said and done, maintaining a tantalizing and fulfilling sexual relationship comes down to embracing who you are, inside and out, so that you can be your best with your partner—emotionally, physically, intellectually, and sexually. I once heard someone say, "If you're looking for love, try looking in the mirror." The confidence that you have in yourself will exude into your relationship with your partner. When you pamper him and make him first in your life, he'll love you for it and will try his best to show you just how much. It comes down to keeping sex sexy! It's important to stay in the game and stay in the proverbial "bedroom" as much as possible. Keep those ideas of closeness, sensuality, and romance at the forefront of your relationship, no matter where you are—bring the bedroom mentality with you wherever you go. Make time to make love frequently! Studies have shown that the more you "do it," the more you want to "do it." So even when your sex drive seems low, go ahead and consider saying yes anyway. You don't have to wait until you're aroused to have sex or make love; allow your partner's touches, kisses, and soft caresses to turn you on and help get you in the mood. If you always wait until you're aroused to get started, you may miss out on a lot of special intimate moments and steamy romance with your partner.

Embrace who you are, and venture out from beneath the security of sheets and clothing so you and your partner can embark together on experiences inside and outside the bedroom that will heighten and deepen your relationship. Behind closed doors, be the girl he wants to "date," the girl that nobody knows but him; and when in public, portray the beautiful, strong woman he wants to marry and show to the world. Step up your game and be everything he wants and needs in a partner. Embrace your beauty, overcome your intimacy inhibitions, and communicate what you want while allowing your partner to do the same. Discover your "nudeness," and unveil all your relationship has in store. *Remember:* Keep a five-inch pair of sexy stilettos under the bed … just in case!

Risqué Truth: The element of surprise should never be far from thought. Spontaneity recreates freshness in your relationship and renews the libido.

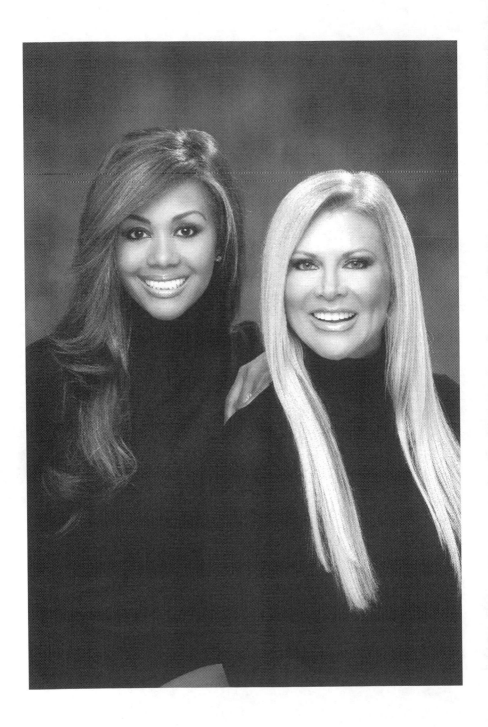

There are some who live in a dream world, and there are some who face reality; and then there are those who turn one into the other.

Douglas Everett

About the Authors

Kym Jackson

Kym's interest in pageants began during college, and in 1986, her first win came when she was crowned First Runner Up in the Miss Texas USA pageant. Since then, Kym was crowned Mrs. Texas United America 2005 and Mrs. Texas 2007 (National Mrs. Pageant), as well as Third Runner Up for Mrs. United America. She currently holds the title of United America Ambassador.

After receiving a BA in Fashion and Fine Arts in 1986, Kym worked at a fashion design house and had the opportunity to use her unique talents designing clothing from 1998 to 2000. Kym's entrepreneurial spirit has made her a successful businesswoman and she has owned day spas, clothing boutiques, and salons across the country; she hosted a talk show; and has been a make-up artist for videos and photo shoots for various clients. She is also a licensed cosmetologist and medical aesthetician. Jackson's first book, on manners and etiquette was written with her daughter, Chauncey, and her mother, Elouise Jackson Beaird. *Powder Puff Principles: Enhancing Your Personal Radiance*, is a generational collaboration that remembers the grace and good manners our mothers and grandmothers displayed in the way they dressed, the way they behaved, and the image they projected. On the heels of that book came *Gentlemen's Principles: A Little Black Book of Etiquette.*

Kym volunteers with the Locks of Love and The Rose Ribbon Foundation, which provide reconstructive surgery to cancer survivors with fixed or low incomes. Other volunteer work includes The Bonita House of Hope, Autism Speaks Foundation, and Yellowstone Academy.

Kym also enjoys playing golf, jogging, and arts and crafts. She resides in Houston, Texas, and she and her husband, Willard L. Jackson have three children - Chauncey, Will, and Blake.

Theresa Roemer

B eauty and fitness pioneer Theresa Roemer is proof that women can have it all! A successful entrepreneur with more than thirty years experience, Theresa continues to think outside the box and has an impressive list of accomplishments to prove it. Her insights in the fitness industry make Theresa a highly sought-after personal trainer. She has previously owned and operated her own health club and mentored young girls on fitness and nutrition through the highly acclaimed Barbizon Modeling Schools. Additionally, her fitness talents have been utilized by one of the top two fitness chains in America.

As well as holding the title of Mrs. Texas United America 2010, and recently winning First Runner Up at the Mrs. United America 2010 pageant, Theresa also won Most Photogenic, People's Vote Online and People's Vote Audience in both of these pageants. She placed in various fitness and bodybuilding competitions between 1990 and 1999, and holds the bodybuilding titles of Miss Wyoming 1999 and Miss U.S. Open 1999. She is co-owner of an energy company, a certified personal trainer, a certified sport nutritionist, a licensed real estate agent, and serves on the board of directors for several entities. She also is an active spokesperson for the American Lung Cancer Association, Texas Children's Hospital, and various other associations and organizations nationwide.

Theresa relentlessly donates her time to various committees and charities at the local, national and international level and truly believes that the biggest thrill and reward in life is to *give*.

One platform very dear to Theresa is Child Legacy International, a non-profit relief organization that seeks to change the face of Africa from despair to destiny by increasing the quality of life and self-sufficiency through the development of sustainable programs.

Theresa is married to Houston businessman Dr. Lamar Roemer, and together they have six children and four grandchildren